HELLO DEARS

HELLO DEARS

MILINDA ROSE ATALLIAN

Library of Congress Control Number:		2010914183
ISBN:	Hardcover	978-1-4535-8408-8
	Softcover	978-1-4535-8407-1
	Ebook	978-1-4535-8409-5

This book was printed in the United States of America.

To order additional copies of this book, contact:
Xlibris Corporation
1-888-795-4274
www.Xlibris.com
Orders@Xlibris.com
87430

CONTENTS

This book is dedicated to Reagan Rose Atallian, my greatest gift. I will always be your Mommy, and you will always be my daughter. My love for you is true, unconditional, and everlasting.

May 1—I found out that I was pregnant.

May 3—I discovered the lump.

May 4—I saw my OBGYN.

May 5—I saw the Breast Surgeon for an exam.

May 11—I had a biopsy done.

May 22—I found out that I had Breast Cancer.

June 4—I found out that we had another miscarriage.

June 9—I had a D&C.

June 26—I had a double mastectomy with reconstructive expanders placed.

. . . and that's pretty much how it started—my journey with Breast Cancer.

Allow me to go back into this list of dates and explain a bit, before I share my Hello Dears with you . . . which will fill you in on some of the many happenings of my story.

I would do the whole, "let me tell you about myself" type of thing, but you will learn enough about who I am by delving into the words of this book. You will get to know me through the love and care that I continue to receive from the people that I surround myself with. I am so fortunate to share my life with them.

My husband Jason and I had been trying to get pregnant for a few months prior to all of "this". We had been seeing our fertility specialist to help us discover when I was ovulating, so we could slip one through the wickets one more time. My fertility and all that goes along with it, could potentially fill another book. The short of it is, I had trouble sustaining pregnancies in the past. At least, before our Reagan Rose came along. We had 5 losses prior to Reagan, so you can imagine how much we treasure our little girl.

The news that we were pregnant was thrilling, especially because we had such a good experience all the way through with Reagan. So, we were excited and optimistic about another little bundle of joy coming into our world.

I am sharing this with you because I believe to my core, that our little bundle who never came to be here on earth, was what lead me to check my ta-ta's that night. I had never been a regular "checker" before. But, something compelled me to circle 'round the little lady lumps to make sure I was OK. Well, it turns out, I wasn't.

Initially, when I discovered the lump, I was reassured that it could just be glandular because I was pregnant. That may have been the best thing that I was told . . . that, and not to worry. That being written, deep down I knew, I just knew.

I am a strong person, but I do worry about things. So, when the Doctor's told me not to . . . I did my best not to. I have to say that throughout this entire process, I haven't . . . worried that is.

Because we were told not to worry, and because we were told that it could be glandular, after I was sent for the biopsy, I went back for the follow up appointment by myself. At that time, I was about 6 weeks pregnant.

I should have known when the Dr. walked in the room, and asked if I had anyone with me, that there was something "wrong". The Dr. looked right at me and said, "I am sorry Milinda, your results did not come back the way we had anticipated, you have carcinoma in your left breast."

The only thing that I could get out of my mouth was, "OK". I took a few deep breaths and then moved on to, "what do I need to do". From that moment until now and forever more, I continue to "do", and I don't intend to stop, not now, not ever.

My Dears

When I first found out that I had Breast Cancer, I immediately felt for my daughter, my husband and my family. I am a fortunate woman, not just because I am a Survivor, but because I share my life with genuine people who love me unconditionally for who I am. I have been told that I am loyal to a fault when it comes to my family and friends. To me, that is an oxymoron . . . one can never been too loyal.

Immediately I wanted to comfort my family, my friends, my "dears" and everyone that would be upset by my news. I wanted to let them know that I was OK, that my family was OK, and that everything was going to be OK despite the shocking revelation. That was my concern during those initial moments after I was told.

I knew that I was going to fight it, I knew that I had found it early and I knew that I was going to Kick It's Ass . . . so, to me, the important thing was to let my family know that I was OK and not to worry. If they threw in some prayers along the way . . . well, that would be fantastic too . . . but truly, I just didn't want them to waste their energies worrying about me.

How was I going to reach out to the many, many people that Jason and I consider to be our family? I didn't want to be on the phone taking up precious minutes reiterating time and time again to everyone that we love, what was going on. I have a friend and former coworker that had battled Breast Cancer just a year prior to my journey . . . and she gave me the wonderful idea of sharing my thoughts and information via email.

Now, to some, email is "cold". I can understand that to an extent. To me, it's an awesome way to keep in touch with people that we care about. Sometimes, people are far more comfortable sharing thoughts via email rather than in person or over the phone . . . I happen to be one of these people. Written words can be read, reread, digested and then read again. You can't do that in person. Don't get me wrong—I will hug and kiss your face, and you will know just how much I care when you are in my company. But, sometimes I don't have the time to do that, so email is a way of quickly letting people know that I am thinking of them. For me, it has been perfect.

When I started sharing my journey through these emails, I went with the notion, that if I had their email address in my address book on our computer, then they knew me well enough to know what our family was going through. So, I went with that. Some people have been added to that list, and some taken away, but each and every person that remains are special, important, and loved by me and my family. They are My Dears, and there is no better way for me to encompass each salutation to each of the people in my life, than "Hello Dears".

So, let me share my journey with you, through the emails that I've written. I will peek in from time to time, to add to my story, and then again at the end to of course say . . . well, you'll just have to skip ahead, or keep reading to get to the end.

Before you begin, I want to thank you for reading my words. They have healed me in ways that are unexplainable.

I also want to say, that as we all very well know, everyone's journey with the "c-word" as I call it, is different. I am in no way suggesting that what I have chosen to do, as far as the treatment of my Breast Cancer is the best way to go. It was my way and still is. It was not without thought, it was not without research, it was not without discussions with my husband and loved ones. It was however, my way. If you should ever know anyone who happens to be diagnosed with Breast Cancer, they too will have their own story to tell and their own "way". Listen to them, learn from them, and then make the best choice that is right for you in your moment with whatever you are dealing with at the time.

CHECK THOSE TA-TA'S

Hello Dears,

If you are getting this email from me, its because you are in my address book. If your in my address book it's because I care about you, and I know you care about me. And since that is the case, I wanted to share our story with you as I wouldn't want you to hear it from anyone else but me.

I know that I haven't been in touch with some of you since the "discovery", so I wanted to send an email to let you all know what is going on.

First and foremost, I want to Thank You, every single one of you, who already know some of what has been taking place, and has shown my family your support. We are so very fortunate to be blessed with a tremendous amount of love and care from our family, our friends, and our neighbors. I can not express to you just how much that means to me/us.

I will keep this as short as possible, knowing that time is precious, but also knowing that sometimes it helps to understand and know what is and will be going on in the next few weeks.

About 6 weeks ago, I went to bed a little earlier than Jason and for some crazy reason, gave myself a breast exam. I can tell you that I have only done this 2-3 other times in my lifetime. So it is amazing to me, that somehow I was lead to do one recently. I discovered a lump on my left side.

Now, I think we can all safely say without hesitation, and with no offense taken, that I am not the largest chested woman in the world:) Finally, finally, this has worked to my advantage! I called my OBGYN and was seen the next morning. She then referred me to a Breast Surgeon at the Breast Center. As I know some of my family members have asked, and some will want to know, I will give you a name of all the Doctor's (at the end of this email) so that you will know who I am seeing. Anywho, they did a biopsy and the results came back . . . well, with not so great news. The lump is cancerous or as they say—I have a carcinoma—in my left breast. Shocking I know.

I can tell you that the nurse and Dr. both said that "You saved your life by finding this lump". So, if there was or is ever any reason for you to grope your tata's, do it now. Do it for me. Have your husband do it. Have your sister or a friend do it. I'll do it if you want, just DO IT!

Anyway, that was on a Tuesday morning, so of course, we all know . . . after Jason, who did I call? My awesome sister, my best girl-friend, Lis. She got on a plane the next day and was here for my round-table appointment with my team of Doctors on Thursday morning. It was so amazing to have her there for support, and to shed her ever-optimistic light on the situation.

Their recommendation is for me to have mastectomy done to remove my left breast. At the same time, they will do a lymph node test to make sure that "it" hasn't spread to my lymph nodes. The Doctor's said that there is a 80% chance that the lymph nodes will be clear . . . meaning that no further treatment will be necessary. It would be so wonderful if that is the case. We will know about a week after the surgery if that is so. If it does come back positive, then we will re-evaluate at that time, and they will recommend radiation and possibly chemotherapy. I am truly hoping that I do not need that—but one day at a time.

One of the reasons they did not recommend a lumpectomy is because I am so small chested . . . the lump that they would be removing, and the placement of the lump, would leave me with a really funky shaped boobie, so off with the whole thing it is!

They also did a blood test at the time of the appointment on Thursday. It's called a BRCA1&2 test. This will determine if I carry the gene that would suggest that I could get the same thing in the other breast and/or ovaries. If I don't, that would be great as well. If I do, then I will be opting to have the other breast removed, so as to be proactive and not have to worry about the cancer arriving in my right breast. They will have the result of that blood test back before my upcoming surgery, so that if need be, they can do a double mastectomy instead of a single. Nothing like getting it all done in one fell swoop!

For that reason, there is also a plastic surgeon on my "team" of Docs. She will be there on the day of the surgery to re-build my breast and/or breasts with implants. That is a good thing because I will not have to go for any period without anything on my chest.

Over the next few weeks, I will be meeting with the plastic surgeon, the oncologist, the radiologist, a psychologist, and some other key docs . . . just to monitor everything, and make sure my mind is right before the big procedure. These are all the Docs that were present at the round-table appointment, along with the Breast Surgeon, that will be performing the mastectomy. Jason, Lis and

I all feel very comfortable with their plan of action for me to get rid of, and do as much as we can to keep the cancer gone.

My sister also spoke with a Dr. up at Thomas Jefferson (which is where she and her husband went to med-school). We faxed her the report from my biopsy, and Lis went over the initial plan of the mastectomy and lymph node test. That Dr. also concurred with treatment. We also talked with Joe's (Lis' husband's) father, who is an oncologist down in Atlanta, about the discovery and treatment plan. He also agreed that it was a great plan of action and is pleased with things thus far.

While it is never easy to discover cancer—especially on yourself—I have a lot of good things going for me where my case in concerned. I found it early. It is treatable. I am young and in good health. The "numbers" with regard to the cancer (ie, HER-2), and the levels of progesterone and estrogen present in the lump are all good things as far as having breast cancer goes. As foreign as this must sound to some of you, just know that I am very fortunate—as fortunate as one can be—in this given predicament.

As shocking as this news was and is, those of you that know me well will understand when I say that: I would much rather be the one that has the cancer, than a member of my family. Having said that, I know that this news will upset some of you even more than it is upsetting for me to have to deal with.

It will be a chore, it will be work, it will be a challenge. It won't be painless, and it will be both overwhelming and exhausting at times. However, I will fight this with everything that I have in order to live a long, vibrant and healthy life. I am extremely positive and will remain so throughout this process. I am sure to have my moments, but I want you all to know that I am OK. Jason and I are OK. Reagan is OK. We will deal with this and continue to be the strong family that we are because we love one another so very much.

We all know the old saying that "Everything happens for a reason" . . . I can't say that I am all the way enamored with that saying at the present moment, but it is true. I believe that there is some reason as to why this is happening to me. I hope that all of you can find your own reason—whether it be to make more time for yourself, to make more time for others, to not take time, health or loved ones for granted, to put "smaller" issues into perspective, to make our Faith stronger, to stop wasting energy on things that do not effect our daily lives, to hug our loved ones closer, to show more affection, to show more sympathy and empathy, to be more open to more things . . . the list is endless. I hope that—in the very least—outside of checking your ta-ta's, that my "story" will persuade you to take some time out and come up with your own reason as to why you think this is happening, and how you can use it to effect your own life in a positive way.

I can tell you that for me, partially, I will be trying very hard every single day, to not worry so much about things beyond my immediate core. A huge task for me I know—and there will be other lessons learned for me when this is all said and done I am sure, but that is part of why I think this may be occurring . . . so that I can let some of the worrying go, focus on myself a bit more, and continue to build our strong, healthy, loving family. I am so very lucky to have the most loving husband in the world. He is not only my husband, but he is my very best friend and the most awesome Daddy to our Reagan Rose. They are my heart and soul, and part of what makes me, me. So again, take some time to gain some kind of lesson out of this crazy scenario of mine . . . please!

My surgery is scheduled for June 26th. Between now and then I shouldn't need much from everyone/anyone except a big squeeze when you see me, along with one for my husband and daughter as well. Once the surgery is done, I will surely let you know what—if anything—I/we need from any of you in terms of help. Let me repeat the last sentence because I know most of you know how private I am and how I tend to like to take care of myself and my family . . . . But, I/we will ask for your help, we will ask for your help when we need it. I/we will not be shy about asking. And if there are periods of time when we are not asking, please know its not because we feel as if we can't, its just because we are truly doing OK.

Again, that being said, hugs are always welcome, along with words, emails, and messages of support.

I will be in touch again, once the surgery takes place to let you know the outcome of the lymph node testing. For now, please pray for me that it will come back "clear", so that no further treatment will be necessary. And . . . once again . . . tell your Moms, your sisters, your daughters, your friends, your co-workers, your neighbors, your girlfriends, your loved ones to check themselves. Feel those ta-ta's! Lube em' up, and make a party out of it. Do it in the shower. Do it at the gym. Do it on the beach. Just do it:) And then go buy something pink:)

My Love To You All,

Milinda

Brigade of Pink

I am not sure of the exact date as to when the Pink started to stream in, but I would say probably between the end of May and the end of June. It was as if someone from Heaven opened up a gigantic bottle of Pepto-bismol and lathered us with it, from head to toe.

Everything Pink that you can imagine, from shoes, to socks, to pj pants, to shorts, a plethora of t-shirts, bikinis, bracelets, hats, scarves, purses, and my personal favorite—pink Gucci sunglasses from my big sister.

Save the ta-ta's, Save Second Base, I wear Pink for my—Wife/Sister/ Daughter, Fight Like a Girl, Live Strong, One Brave Chic, and so on and so on and so on. I received so many nice gifts, with the appropriate triumphant—Pink color—it was fantastic!

We were swimming in Pink. Some pink ribbon items were in the mix as well, but if it was Pink, we had it . . . and so did our immediate family members!

In some ways, I think that the Pink paraphernalia served as some sort of comfort. If we wrapped ourselves in Pink, then everything would be OK.

I have talked to many women who still wear Pink proudly, whether it be for themselves, or in honor of someone that they love.

I have also talked to Survivors who don't wear a stitch of it. As a matter of fact, one of the nurses that took care of me in the recovery room, who is a Survivor, said "I won't wear Pink for the rest of my life" . . . . I guess she got sick of the bubble-gum hue!

The point is; I was covered in Pink, and still wear it proudly. I understand that some women don't want to wear it, and I understand why some women don't like to participate in Breast Cancer functions, fundraisers and events. Truly I do. I get it. They lived through it, and now they are done . . . but ladies, are we ever really done? I think not.

When you have Survived something as gripping as Breast Cancer, no matter what your journey entailed, it changes you. So I say, buy that Pink stuff and sport it like a champion.

6-12-09

Save the Ta-ta's

Hello Dears,

I wanted to give you all a brief update as to what has been going on, and what will be taking place in the next couple of weeks/months. First and foremost, I would like to sincerely Thank You, for all of your hugs, calls, emails, messages, cards and words of support. I can't begin to express to you how much the outpouring of thoughtfulness means to Jason, Reagan and myself. It isn't always easy to know what to say when someone tells you news such as mine, but somehow each of you has found a way to make us feel loved and cared for in this situation. I have kept all of your emails in a file called "Kick it's Ass", and when need be, I re-read them for inspiration.

We continue to be strong and positive as we head into the treatment portion of this journey. Now that all of the "discovery" (as my sister called it) is done, we are geared up and ready to deal with the surgery.

The good news that has come out of the past couple of weeks . . . along with me catching the "c-word" early, is that my gene test came back negative. The BRCA1&2 are negative, which means that I am not a gene carrier for this cancer. Our Reagan, along with my sister and her girls, do not have to be concerned that the cancer is in our bloodlines. I cannot tell you how huge that is for me. To know that the family members who are nearest and dearest to my heart, need not worry about this over their lifetimes, is a relief to say the least. That's not to say that they won't be proactive in checking their ta-ta's, because they certainly will be . . . as will you and yours!

I am opting to have a double mastectomy along with a right nipple-save. Because the right side is my "healthy" side, the plastic surgeon will be able to save my "nip" and use it on my new set! This will also give her something to compare the new left side to when she is building it.

Three things will happen during my surgery:

First, they will be doing a lymph-node check. This is the test that we are all praying for to come back negative. The results from that test will be back a week or so after the surgery.

Second—"off with their heads". Dr. Dickson-Witmer will be removing my breast tissue on both sides. She will be chucking everything except for the right nipple:)

Last—but not least—Dr. Banbury (the plastic surgeon) will be putting in expanders on both sides. This word makes it seem like there will be some type of metal building going on . . . but please rest assured—I will not be sporting head-gears on my boobies, the expanders are plastic round circles that will be going underneath my skin. They are shaped like an implant, and will look like breasts. They will not feel like a breast however . . . As she explained it, they will feel more like "rocks". My good friend Sharon (a SURVIVOR-yipee!) also described them as "turtle shells" . . . lovely. These expanders will stay in for approximately 2-3 months. I will be getting them filled weekly until they get to be the size that I am happy with. No, there will not be holes in my chest . . . they use a stud-finder (I'm serious) to find the place where a small needle will go in, to fill the "humps". The Dr. assured me, that if able, I can workout and even run with them in. They won't "give" like the final set, but I can still get a sweat going, so that is great news for me.

Barring any further treatment, once the expanders are filled-up (to the size that I like), I will then have a final surgery to have the expanders out and the silicone implants in. This second surgery is apparently a lot less uncomfortable than the first one.

Speaking of which—The week or two following surgery will be the most uncomfortable. I will be very sore from the procedures and not be able to move around much. They will be putting drains in both sides, for the first few days. This will help to alleviate the pressure from the fluids building up. They will also have a morphine pump attached to me for those first few days. I am a quick healer and have a high tolerance for pain, so I don't anticipate being in too much pain after the first few weeks. However, I know that I will not be as "on the go" as I am now while recovering. I plan to take it as easy as possible during the recovery period.

We are having a cleaning lady come in once a week (for two months) to help with house cleaning. Jason is taking off the first couple of weeks to help me and to help with Reagan. My Mom will also be here—as needed—to help. And, Lis will be in and out of town during those first few weeks/months after my surgery. Brian is going to help us with cutting the grass, and we have a plan in place for help with meals. Jason has also been given a month-long pass to the Y. This came as a huge relief to me because it will allow him to get routine work-outs in, and also allow Reagan to visit with her friends in her "room" at the Y. It will give them both a break, while keeping some sort of normalcy during the weeks following my surgery.

My surgery will be at Wilmington Hospital on June 26th. I have to be there at 6am, and the surgery will start at 8. I am not sure how long the procedures will take, but once they are done, I will ask Jason to let his Mom know that I am OK and that they are done. I will then be asking Jason's Mom to contact you—via email—to let you know that I am OK and on the road to recovery. I would expect this to come sometime in the afternoon on the 26th. If you are at all worried, or need to know before you hear from her (and I understand if that is the case), Jason will have his cell phone on, as well as my Dad, and my sister. I will give you their numbers at the end of this email. You can call them to see what's up if you can't wait for the email.

We are going to be leaving for our vacation with my Mom, and Alissa's family next Saturday the 20th. We are headed to our usual spot in Kiawah, SC. It will be so nice to get away for a bit, before all of this takes place. I will be taking it easy, but also enjoying our family and getting my normal work-outs in before the big day. We will be returning on the 25th in the afternoon, so that we can all get set for the next morning.

We have a good plan in place that both Jason and I are comfortable with in terms of taking care of Reagan, not only the day of, but the weeks following until I am able to take care of her without help. Again, if we need any extra hands, I know that I can ask any of you, and you will be here to help out. I will do so if need be, we will do so if need be. If we aren't asking . . . once again . . . just know that it is because we are doing OK, and are taking care of business over here in Brookmeade:)

Once I am able to, after the surgery takes place, I will be in touch again. And we will certainly let you know about the node testing when we get those results.

For now, and until then, we are going to keep taking things one day, and one step at a time. I will keep squeezing these freakin' lemons that are being catapulted my way, into lemonade . . . w/ a little splash of American Honey! I am in full-fighters-mode to kick this c-words ass, so no worries, its almost outt-a-here!

I am so truly lucky to have all of your support, and the support of my loving husband, my incredible daughter, and our family. Love is a full-circle expression, and I can tell you that for as much love as I have given over my years . . . and we all know that I know how to give out the lovin' . . . it has come back to me in-full from all of you. Keep the prayers coming, along with the positive thoughts and good vibes. We will all get through this together and come out stronger than ever. We'll just have a hell of a lot more pink items to wear when we are done!

My Love to you all,

Milinda

WHY THE DOUBLE?

I think that now would be an appropriate time for me to share why I chose to have a double mastectomy, rather than a single.

When I was first diagnosed, the Doctor's recommended a single mastectomy rather than a lumpectomy—for a few reasons. The first reason was because I was pregnant at the time, and could not receive radiation, if needed, after the surgery. If I were to have a lumpectomy, it would have been followed up with radiation treatment of that area. The second reason was that my ta-ta's were so ta-ta-teeny-tiny to begin with, that the lumpectomy would have left me, well, lumpy looking.

Once I had the miscarriage, the option for the lumpectomy was revisited, but I had already wrapped my brain around the mastectomy, and wasn't going to change it back. I knew that I wanted my ta-ta gone, so that the c-word had no place to come back to.

After meeting with the plastic surgeon, I decided to go with the double mastectomy, again for a few reasons. The first being, I did not want the c-word to invade my other ta-ta. The second was, that I wanted everything to be even. I didn't want sensation in one side and not the other—that would have driven me crazy. The appearance would be much more appealing with both sides being the same. So, I was confident in my decision to have them both removed. "Off with their heads."

I continue to be happy with my choice, not only because the Dr. did find another lump forming, that would not have been removed with an initial lumpectomy; but I am also confident that the c-word is now gone and has no ta-ta to come back to.

I understand that, to some, this decision was radical. However, I am a young woman, who happens to take really good physical care of myself. I was confident that I would heal quickly and be on the path back to my healthy lifestyle despite the major surgery.

Everyone has to make decisions with regard to their health at one point or another. My decision worked well for me. That's not to say that it would have worked for someone else. For me, I wanted to be in control of things, and start anew, with some new ta-ta's on board!

6-25-09

Boob-Voy-Age'

Hello Dears,

Well, we are home from our vacation. It was amazing and awesome as usual. Time spent with those that you love always is, and always should be. This time was no exception. We enjoyed the beach, as well as the pool—and of course the golf was "fantastic". Watching our girls play and laugh with each other is something that would make anyone forget anything that is troublesome, so I am glad that we were able to get away and be together.

Now that we are home, and settled in, we are gearing up for our day tomorrow.

It goes without saying, but I will say it again anyway . . . I care for and love each and every one of you. I am so lucky to have you in my life. We are so lucky to be able to share our daily joys, our accomplishments, our good times and some of our bad with you. I feel so blessed to have your love and support. It means the world to us. So, get your prayers stretched out and ready to rock tomorrow morning.

Once I am out of the OR, and Jason has a chance to see my face, he will call his Mom.

I hope to be home the next day (Saturday) from the hospital. My sister is coming into town on Saturday and will be here into the following week to make sure that I am recovering well.

As soon as I am able, I will send you an email to let you know that things are moving along well and that I am healing up like a champ.

I mentioned before that it will be harder for my Jason, Mom, Dad, Sister and their Loved ones to have to wait for me while I am in the OR, so please say some prayers for strength for them as well.

As I was enjoying one of my runs in Kiawah on the beach, I looked out onto the ocean and saw a group of dolphins. They seemed to be following me along the way. Tears came to my eyes, as I felt their unknowing support. I watched them dive down, resurface, and dive down again. They followed me for almost four miles, and I watched them the entire time. When I finished my run, I stood at the foot of the ocean. My Asics were at the edge of the water. I closed my eyes and let the waves and sand rush over my shoes. The tide rushed in and out, just like its suppose to. Now, anyone that owns a good pair of running shoes will tell you how much they covet their kicks. I bare no exception to this rule, but that day, I let the ocean water and the sand run over my feet again and again. The water, the tide, and ALL that is beyond—all of my loved ones, from the past and the present, and all of our ANGELS were gripping onto the "bad", taking it out to sea, and replacing it with more strength (as if I didn't have enough) but, more strength came with each passing wave. More "bad" was taken away and more "good" was brought in with each break. It was surreal, it was beautiful, it was a moment in time that I will never forget. Just me, the ocean, the good coming in and the bad being washed away. I am ready now.

I will be OK. Jason and I will be OK. Jason, Reagan and I will be OK. Our family will be OK. Everything is going to be all-right. I believe this to be true, I have Faith that this will be true. Its time for me to KICK SOME SERIOUS ASS. This c-word will be met with a fury that it cannot and will not be able to handle. I will be tired along the way, there will be moments of wonder and frustration, I may be scared and hurting at times, but I have all of you to lean on. You will give me the strength that I will need to get through and endure whatever lies ahead. I have so much to live for. I love my husband and my daughter more than I could ever begin to describe—they forever own my heart and soul. I have been given the gift of the best Mom, and the most loving Dad in the whole world. My Sister has been and will continue to be my rock, she is the truest meaning of the words BIG SISTER. Jason and I have a handful of ANGELS that will be looking out for me during this surgery and the next . . . and all that comes in between. For all of these people just mentioned, and the ANGELS as well, I WILL BE OK.

Keep Me,
My Love to You All,

Milinda

July 2, 2009

☺

Hello Dears,

Well, I am one week out from the Boob-voy-age', and I am doing great! The surgery itself went very well, and my recovery thus far has been quick. That's not to say that I am moving too quickly or pushing myself, b/c I am not . . . but I am recovering at a speedy little pace.

My hospital experience was fantastic, everyone treated me very well, especially the nurses—every single one. Apparently I asked for a shot of tequila (which I have never had), and some *serenity now*, when the nurses asked me if I needed anything! This is exceptionally funny because the nurse's name was Jerry . . . . And we are huge Seinfeld fans. I am sure if you are as well, you will easily recall the serenity now episode. Jason and I were in stitches (no pun intended)!

My sister came into town the day after surgery and left on Wednesday afternoon. Between Jason, Alissa, my Mom, and my Dad & Susan, we had all kinds of help with me, and with Reagan. I can't ever thank them enough for all that they have done and will do as I keep on pounding through this journey.

W/o going into too much detail, the surgeon's work is spectacular. You cannot tell that I had anything done . . . except for the stitches and bandages. The size of the expanders (for now:)) are the same size as my old "set", so when I look down, that is what I see.

Lis helped me shower, and change the bandages the day after I got home. I was able to wash my hair, and the next day able to do the same and shave. It was so incredibly reassuring to have her stay here and make sure that things were looking "OK". When she did leave for South Carolina on Wednesday, Jason and I both felt confident that I was mobile enough to begin taking care of myself on my own. Again, that's not to say that I will be pushing the lawn mower around as I normally do . . . but I am able to move about w/o anyone telling me to sit back down—and that has a lot to do with Lis being here. Alissa is an angel on earth to me. (sniff, sniff)

It would take me too long to tell you all that everyone has done for me/us so far, but believe me when I tell you that I am cared for, thought of, prayed for, taken care of, appreciated, loved, and so much more that I can't put into words. All of them, and all of you are wonderful. And my Jason, and Reagan are a constant source of inspiration. They are healing me with each and every smile—they are my medicine. (sniff, sniff—again . . . sorry ☺)

Now, onto the treatment: They did find a "teensy-tiny" fragment in my centinal node, so she went in and tested some other nodes to see what's up.

This news was a tad startling as we kind of expected everything to be clear (remember the 80% statement)?! . . . well, we all know me right? Right. So, Dr. Dickson-Witmer tested 8 more nodes at the time of the surgery. We had our appointment today to see what is going on with the other nodes . . . . The first thing the Dr. said when she entered the room was "Milinda, I have good news". I had thought for a fleeting moment that she was in the wrong room, but since she said my name, the moment passed and she began to talk. All of the rest of my nodes are CLEAR! CLEAR! CLEAR! and CLEAR!

That is fantastic. Here comes some medical jargon, so bare with it . . . . The fragment that was present in the cent. node was, as she said, teeny-tiny. If there is enough "material" (fragment) to send out, they will send it for an onco-type-dx test. If that test occurs, it will determine whether or not chemotherapy is necessary. If there is not enough "material" (because the fragment is so small), than Dr. Wozniak (the oncologist), will determine what course of action would be best for my treatment. Because of my age (young for breast cancer), Dr. Dickson-Witmer, seemed to think that he may lean towards one round of chemotherapy, but she didn't say definitively. I have an appointment with Dr. Wozniak on July 10th in the afternoon. We will know my course of action after that appointment and what lies ahead.

Dr. Dickson Witmer said again that "you saved your life", the right breast was "clear"—meaning there was no cancer in that one . . . its off with their heads anyway. The left side however had the cancer-lump in it that I felt, as well as another one forming in the secondary tissues. So, once again, I am, we are, everyone is, so glad that I found the lump and caught this early on.

Once we get the report from Dr. Wozniak, and hear his treatment plan, we will once again run it by Joe's Dad, and the Dr. up at Jefferson, to make sure they concur. We are so lucky to have them for second and third opinions.

For now, we will keep taking one day at a time, and continue to Thank GOD, for each other, for you, and for everyone and anyone that has been touched by this crazy-ass—c-word. I will be in touch once we see Dr. Wozniak and let you know what is going to happen. In the mean time, I expect to see Dr. Banbury for her to check out my expanders and see that they are healing up as expected. All is well, I am OK, Jason is OK, Reagan is OK, we are all doing great.

Thank you all, again for your constant support, I can feel it. Truly I can. Keep em' coming. Keep wearing pink proudly. And, please, don't forget to tell any and every woman in your life that you care about . . . to CHECK THOSE Ta-Ta's!

My Love to You All,

Milinda

Don't Ask ... Just Do

So, here is a little piece of advice ... or rather an observation that I now practice myself. I wanted to pass it along to you, because I realize that when loved ones are faced with the supportive predicament, sometimes its hard to know what to do, or say.

I happen to be somewhat of a private person, when it comes to certain things. I like to take care of myself, and my family on my own. That is what gives me pleasure and satisfaction. All of My Dears know this about me.

That being said, if someone were to ask me if I needed anything, my general answer would be "No, Thank you". And, that is usually because I don't or didn't need any help.

OK, so THAT being said, sometimes the best thing to do for yourself and for your loved one is to just *DO*. Don't ask, just do.

If you want to do something for someone that is struggling with something, just do it. Send them a card, send an email, send them a handwritten note, or leave them a kind message, just to let them know you are thinking of them. Make them a meal and drop it off, or make them something sweet to indulge in. Take them some vino, or their Starbucks drink of choice.

Whatever it is that would make you feel like you put a smile on their face ... just do it.

Don't ask them if you can, or you should, or if they want you to, just DO IT!

It's the best way to let them know you care, and to appease the thoughtful urge within you to take care of someone that you love.

Don't ask ... just do ... believe me, your act of kindness will come back to you.

In the Mean Time, Think Pink

Hello Dears,

The ties that bind are vast. They are everlasting, and stretch beyond the horizon; too far to see their ending place—because there isn't one.

In the last two weeks I/we have heard from Family, both near and far. Grandparents, Aunts, Uncles (both near and distant), Cousins (both near and distant), Friends, former co-workers, former employers, Jason's current friends/co-workers, wives of those co-workers, neighbors—both some that we are friends with and some who we know in passing, "pool" friends, daughters and sons of all of the above, and so on, and so on. It has been amazing to say the least.

I wrote this before, but it continues to stand true—All of the love, time, support, attention, tradition, affection, and prayers that I have given, and maintained over the years, has come back to me, and my family . . . overwhelmingly so. I can't tell you enough how much it makes the difference. Words will never begin to express how Thankful I am, and will forever be.

I won't keep you long as the summer months are zooming by, but I did want to let you know what's been going on.

We saw Dr. Banbury (the Plastic Surgeon) on Monday, and she said that I am healing up very well. She "ok'd" me to start working out . . . so we (Jason, myself, Reagan and my Mom) were at the Y the next day! It was nice to see my "y-friends" and get a sweat going. I did the Precor and "walked vigorously" as that is all that I am allowed to do for the next week. Then, if all continues to go well, I can begin to run . . . one step at a time.

I continue to pull myself back from doing too much, and have a few people around me that are doing the same☺ I see Dr. Banbury again on Wednesday for my first "fill". This is when she will use the stud-finder and fill up my expanders a bit at a time, over time, until I get to be the size that I am happy with.

I have been feeling really strong and doing great since the surgery. I am confident it is because I have had Mom and Jason around to help me. Mom has been fantastic with Reagan, and with cooking meals for us as I get myself going again.

Because Reagan is a gift in-and-of herself, Mom too has enjoyed her time with Reagan. I wouldn't have it any other way, and knowing that they are spending time together has made my healing happen that much faster.

Jason will go back to work on Monday. His SWAT team members, as well as other officers have constantly been calling, coming by and emailing him to check up on him, and our family over the past two weeks. The trust that those officers have in each other is as strong as the support that they have shown our family.

I continue to be able to do more each day and will take each day at time to allow myself to do more things.

A special Thank You to my Mom and Jason for the past ten days. I love, honor, and respect you both more each and every day. (sniff-sniff)

So, today we saw the Oncologist (Dr. Wozniak). We had been told that his personality isn't the greatest, but I have to say, that I liked him a lot. He was matter of fact, very informative and most importantly, not "chemo-happy". He went over the pathology report with us and re-informed us that the tissue that was taken out, has many "good" things going for it/me. Being estrogen and progesterone positive, are good things. To keep things short, basically we are waiting for the onco-type test to come back. It will be 2-3 more weeks before it is back. He (Dr. W.) is a firm believer in that test, as am I . . . and Joe's Dad, as well as my sister and her husband.

There are three levels that the test will determine for me/us.

If I am at a Low-level, then he recommends hormonal therapy. This will be pill form, no chemotherapy.

If I am at an Intermediate-level, then he will see where I fall within that range and decide from there, but suggested that he would still lean towards just hormonal therapy, and no chemotherapy.

If I am at a High-level, which he thinks b/c of the pathological information of the tumor tissues, and nodes, then I will need both chemotherapy and hormonal therapy.

He does not want to jump start me on any treatments until the test results are back. I am more than comfortable with that decision. And while it is hard to wait, I am OK with waiting b/c then we will know what course of action is best. If I don't need something, than I certainly don't want to put my body through the ringer, just to do it. The long term effects of things—as far as chemotherapy treatment—are being taken into consideration by him, and I appreciate that.

So, again, we will just have to wait and see. In the mean time, he is happy that I already take good care of myself. I will continue to do that, along with some added Vitamin D, and see him in a few weeks. Right now, my appointment is scheduled for Aug. 31st, but I will be calling his office in two weeks to see if the results are back before then.

During that time, I will be seeing Dr. Banbury for the expander "fills". I will continue to breathe, take one day at a time, and be so very thankful that I found the lump in its early stages.

I will continue to pray for anyone and everyone that has been touched by the "c-word". I will continue to be thankful for each and every one of you. I am so lucky. I still know and believe that I will be OK, no matter what course of action has to be taken, I will be OK.

Keep enjoying your summer. Keep sharing my "story" with anyone that you feel would benefit from hearing it. I want people to know, I want people to be open about it. I want people to check their ta-ta's. I have one more request . . . . Along with a hug the next time you see me . . . please, give someone you love an extra dose of affection. Whether it be your Mother, your Father, your Sister, your Children, another Family Member, a Friend, a co-Worker, a Neighbor, or even someone who looks as if they could use it . . . give them a squeeze . . . do it for and from me.

My Love to You All,

Milinda

7-12-09

THE TIES THAT BIND . . .

Hello Dears,

Just a quick one . . . .
I wanted to share something amazing with you.
A friend of ours named Mico Santos, is a police officer, and works with Jason. He is on the SWAT team, and we have come to care for and respect him a lot over the past 13 years. His wife's name is Ryan. Since the first time I met Ryan (who used to work at Maureen's behind the front desk—and is now working at Barclay's), I told Mico again and again how beautiful she is. And she is. She is tall, blonde, and has a beautiful smile. Moreover, she is kind and always friendly when we see her. Now, I am certain that she is even more beautiful on the inside than she is on the outside . . . .

Ryan participated in her first Avon Breast Cancer walk in San Francisco last year. Mico's sister lives there, and though neither one of them "knew" anyone who has/had Breast Cancer, she decided to join Mico's wife and walked last year.

This year, she wanted to do the same, although now her cause became a bit more personal . . . as she knows me:). She wore my name on the sticker that she walked with during the race. Ryan also signed my name on a huge inflatable Breast Cancer sign at the end of the race. I can't tell you how very moved I am that she had me in mind during her walk this year.

The ties that bind are vast.

I will get a chance to thank her in person this Thursday as there is an upcoming SWAT event that Jason and I are attending. I just wanted to share this part of my "story" with you all, and let you know that there are some really, awesome, and amazing things happening during this journey.

I will send you some pictures as they forward them to me, so you can see for yourself, just how beautiful Ryan Santos is.

My Love to You All,

Milinda

7-23-09

Goldie-Locks

Hello Dears,

I'll just get right to it . . . . I found out today (because I called the lab in CA myself), that I DO NOT NEED chemotherapy!

There isn't a word that can fully encompass the sense of relief that I feel having found that out . . . . Because as you know, or may have come to find out through these e-mails, I am pretty crafty when choosing my words☺

Basically, the onco-type test is complete and I "scored" a 13. On a scale 0-100, 100 being the highest level. I am lucky thirteen!

So, during my very, very brief, and kind-of awkward conversation (only b/c I pushed myself into his office-space today) . . . Dr. Wozniak gave me the numbered results, and told me that he would be recommending hormonal (pill form) therapy. And that chemotherapy would not be recommended for me.

Please turn to the closest window in your house, or office, or wherever you are, and gaze out at the tree leaves blowing . . . That's not the wind, nor mother nature moving those leaves—that is my sigh of relief permeating across Delaware, South Carolina, Pennsylvania, North Carolina, New York, Indianapolis, Maryland, and all of the other states and countries that are lucky enough to hold the homes of those that I love. Yup, that's me, it's a huge sigh that will continuously be active as we turn the corner of this journey.

We have the official meeting with Dr. Wozniak to go over the hormonal treatment plan on the 31st. I will be in touch with you all again after that.

As for the ta-ta's, they are coming along very well. The expanders are uncomfortable, to say the least. But, I am managing, and will keep looking forward to getting them out, and the silicone in. That should happen in the next two months. I will certainly let you know when that surgery will be taking place when we find out. In the mean-time, the (the ta-ta's) are coming along . . . or "are under construction" as I so eloquently put it when people ask me.

I am so thankful for this journey. I am so thankful that I get to keep my Goldie-locks. I am so thankful for all of you, and for all of your support. I am so thankful to be able to give you some good news.

Enjoy your warm summer nights, and I will write again soon, as things keep moving along.

Give each other a squeeze from me . . . just know that when the "real-hug" from me happens . . . if it happens sooner rather than later . . . you'll be hugging some turtle-shells . . . but do squeeze hard, b/c the hugs are part of what heals me.

My Love to You All,

Milinda

"Chicken Empanadas"

. . . Yes Dears,

That is what my loving (and he is very loving) husband refers to my ta-ta's as . . . "the chicken empanadas".

I have to admit, they are shaped like an empanada, although I wish they felt as flexible. These suckers are stationary and do not budge. Still, they are coming along with each weekly "pump-up" session. I am about half way there as far as my desired size goes, so 4 or 5 more sessions, and then I will patiently wait for the silicone-implant-surgery.

I have been running every-other day, and started to lift weights again, so I am keeping things in shape around the mexican-treats☺

I will continue to see Dr. Banbury weekly until I am "full", and then (as I learned today), need to wait 5-6 weeks after the last fill before my final ta-ta surgery. Hmmmm, it seems as if I will be hanging onto the empanadas a little longer than I had anticipated!

As for our appointment w/ Dr. Wozniak today: It went well. He is a tad quirky, but direct and very knowledgeable about his field. I am confident that he has a good plan in place for me. I do have a call out to our OBGYN team, and will wait to hear back from them before I start taking the oral pill that he has prescribed (tamoxifin). I have a few "womanly" and "motherly" questions that I'd like to ask before I start the medicine.

He (Dr. Wozniak) has recommended the normal protocol of a 5 year course of medications—one pill a day—GULP. Joe's Dad agrees with this plan. I will be seeing him every three months for the time being, to check-in and make sure that I am continuing to stay on the cancer-free track. The side effects read like those that you hear on the Viagra commercials (minus the 5 hour erection . . .

ouch)! Everyone is different, so one never knows how my body will react. The side effects are generally mild, so I am not overly worried.

I will keep taking one day at a time and think positively about the prescribed-preventative-pain in my ass-pills☺—And I say that with the best, most empathetic, most understanding, most fortunate, most acutely aware of how lucky I am,—intentions.

Everything else is back to normal, for the most part. Reagan is growing in leaps and bounds. She continues to put a smile on our faces w/ every moment that we spend with her. She makes us aware that life is indeed too precious to waste any energy on things that are stressful. What a beautiful girl Reagan Rose is, she's the best.

Jason is superbly busy back to work. He is on a specialized SWAT team, as well as helping with the Vice President (yes, "Joe") comings and goings in and out of DE. He is also training for a Triathlon in his "free-time", so quite frankly, he is looking better than ever, or as Reagan says. "Daddy is so handsome" . . . . I wonder where she picked that phrase up from?

Our family is doing well, we are still awe struck by the never-ending support, of all kinds, that we have received throughout this journey. Thank you all for all that you do.

As for the "journey", it is not yet over. I am not done fighting. I am still handling things with as much ease as possible, and taking one step at a time. I am uncomfortable and tired at times, but I am here. I am strong, and will continue to stay strong while I fight through and finish out this process . . . however long that takes.

For now, I will be looking forward to getting the empanadas out, so that I can start the healing process after that surgery. I will be a Mommy, a Wife, a Daughter, a Sister, an Aunt, a Granddaughter, a Niece, a Cousin, a Friend, and beyond. You have surrounded me with a strong foundation to lean on, so I will keep on leaning.

I will be in touch over the next few weeks, to let you know how the transformation from empanadas, to a mini-sized bag of jiffy-pop popcorn goes.

Stay cool, give each other a hug from me . . . for now, it will still be a hard-hug, but that's OK, my arms will be open when I see you, so come on in for one!

My Love to You All,

Milinda

8-19-09

Bosu Balls

Hello Dears,

Well, it seems as if I have gone from one analogy to another. That's OK with me, because as much of you know, I thoroughly enjoy a good analogy! For those of you who do not know what a bosu ball is, or may have seen one, but didn't know the name of the apparatus . . . they are half circles, used on the ground for balance, ab workouts and pushups . . . google it and you will see what I mean☺ . . . I went from the "empanadas" to the "Bosu Balls"! Hilarious!

I will tell you this: these ta-ta's of mine are coming along well, but they are as hard as rocks and not all that comfortable. With each "fill" of the expanders, they are getting bigger bit-by-bit, but they are also getting harder. They are not painful, and it's something that I can surely handle for the time being. The expanders are doing a great job stretching my skin out. The best way that I can describe the "fills" and the day or two following, is that someone . . . a really big someone . . . is giving me a bear hug and won't let go. Now, it's a well known fact—that I am all about giving the hugs—however, I do let go eventually . . . un-like the bosu-balls!

I would think that I will get 2 or 3 more fills over the next few weeks and then we will schedule the surgery from there. No worries, I will not be going too big w/ the ta-ta's as I'd like to be able to run w/o the new set getting in the way . . . However, I will be sporting a nice rack when this is all said and done☺

As for the medicine, I started to take that this week. So far so good, so we will keep our fingers crossed that everything will continue to move along with that.

Looking ahead a tad—Get your walking/running shoes ready—The annual 5k for Breast Cancer is being held on my 35th Birthday this year, on October 18th. It will be in Wilmington, around the riverfront area. There will be a run and walk portion of the race. I am planning to run it. I have friends who have participated in the race and have heard how moving it is to be a part of. It will be awesome for me to run this year, and while I may not be logging in my best time, I will be running each step knowing how lucky I am to have come this far, this fast, while still on this journey. It will be amazing to be a part of something local that supports such a great cause. And now, to be counted among the ranks of women who have gone through and are continuing to go through the c-word process, I am sure to be awe-struck.

I am also planning to take the bosu-balls around the DE Distance Run, which is a 15k. That race is the week before the Breast Cancer race, so I will be ready to rock on the 18th . . . and now, you will too because of the advanced notice that you've just been given☺

I will be in touch with you all again soon, to keep you updated on my ta-ta's. I am sure that you'll be eager to find out what Jason's next analogy will be! For the next few weeks we will be getting Reagan ready to start a two-day-per-week program at St. Mary's in the fall, and gearing up for football season . . . go Eagles.

Thank You all for your continued prayers, thoughts, hugs, and words of encouragement to me and our family. Enjoy the last weeks of summer, and . . . if you see a bosu-ball, just remember Jason's comparison, that will surely put a smile on your face.

My Love To You All,

Milinda

9-16-09

A Royale with Cheese

Hello Dears,

Well, I have heard from several of you on my list wanting an update . . . so here's a little one for you as not much has been happening in the last few weeks . . . other than . . . the *EXPANDERS!*

Hmm, I would say that the last couple of weeks have been the most uncomfortable that I have been since the start of this journey. Lack of sleep due to the increasingly hard expanders and just the "feel" of the expanders alone has me feeling—at times—tired and just plain muk-ad! I am getting through for sure, but really really really looking forward to the softer side of silicone:)

I have been going to see Dr. Banbury about once a week to every ten days or so for "fills". She is taking her time w/ the fills to decrease the amount of discomfort . . . oh my! It is hard (no pun intended) to tell what "size" I am per-say . . . yup, I typed per-say. This is b/c the expanders are outbound towards my armpits and not inbound towards my inner chest. The Doc has reassured me that when she does the final surgery, she will release the expanders from my muscle (they are sewn in now) and place the silicone further in towards my chest. That is fantastic news as I surely feel that these things are in my pits! With each fill, they get harder and harder. So, now, I can't sleep on my sides b/c the darn things are in the way . . . and not moving. And, of course I can't sleep on my chest b/c well . . . rocks are in the way!

I feel as if I am complaining so let me just say, once again, how lucky I am to be present and here. And again, how I realize that my path has far less bumps in the road than those traveled by other women. Still, I am freakin' uncomfortable, so I allow myself to say it aloud every once in a while, and then I move onto something else.

As for the medicine . . . as far as I can tell, everything is OK with it. The only side effects that I am experiencing are the hot flashes (very internal, very hot), and a weird desire to eat chalk. No worries, I haven't taken a bite out of any of Reagan's sidewalk chalk as of yet . . . but I do salivate at the thought. I bought a tub-load of Tums at Costco, which seems to be keeping me away from chomping down on the white stuff.

I am still running and getting to the Y, so that makes me feel good. I was planning to run a 15k in mid October, but have decided against it. My sister gently reminded me that I am already pushing my body to do a lot, just by walking around w/ these darn expanders . . . so, to run a longer race just wouldn't be the smartest thing to do. I am sure that the longer races will come again once I am more comfortable and healed.

I am however going to run in the Breast Cancer Race. I know that I mentioned this before, but it is sure to be an emotional day for our family. My plan is to run the race, and then walk w/ some family members who intend to walk the 2.5 mile portion of the mornings event. The "list" of women that I know who have fought this disease continues to grow each and every time I talk with someone. So, I will be running for them. I will be running for their friends, and family who support them in their fight. I will be running for me, for my husband, for our Daughter. I will be running it for the "bun" that lead me to discover the lump, as well as our 6 angels who are shining stars in the heavens. I will be running it for my Mother, for my Father, for my Sister and her Family, and for all of you who have sent your ever-present thoughts of prayer, strength and healing.

I will surely be feeling each color of emotion during my strides . . . from the dark colors filled w/ deep moments of fear, anger, and frustration. Through the blues that hold my tears of pain and of happiness, and the tears of my loved ones. To the brighter colors filled with relief, joy and an abundance of thanks. And finally onto the glorious PINK b/c I am in the process of rounding out my journey, and kicking the c-words ass!

Did I mention that it will be an emotional day? (sniff-sniff)

OK, that should do it for now . . . I will be in touch again soon, with a date for surgery . . . I am wanting to have things done by Turkey Day, so we shall see how the next few weeks shake out.

For now, I will explain the subject-line and then make my way back to my day. "A Royale with Cheese"—for those of you who do not know—is a line from the movie Pulp Fiction. This is how John Travolta's character refers to a BigMac. Can you guess where this is going? No? All-right . . . I went from Chicken Empanadas, to Bosu Balls, and now apparently resemble two "Royales with Cheese"! Imagine that, I haven't eaten red meat in 20 years and now appear to have BigMac's attached to my chest underneath my clothes! Oh my how I love my dear Husband!

Take care, keep wearing Pink, keep the prayers coming and I will write again soon.

My Love to You All,

Milinda

THE CHALK FETISH

Now would be a good time to explain my chalk fetish by saying that there really isn't any explanation for it. Sorry.

Ever since I started to take Tamoxifin, I have had an incredible, unexplainable, unsatisfiable, unwavering craving to eat chalk.

I salivate at the thought of it. I have no idea why, but its stronger than any other urge I have had as far as food cravings go. That is not to say that chalk is a food, its just to say that I have the craving, it hasn't lessened, and I don't anticipate it going away.

Yes, I have discussed my propensity to want to meal on chalk with my team of Doctor's. Most of them have laughed, how could you not?! My plastic surgeon gets a big kick out of it, and went so far as to look it up in one of her many medical references.

There is a condition called PICA, where women (mostly pregnant) want to eat chalk. It's due to lack of one thing or another, but usually goes away after their pregnancies are over.

I can tell you that today, I am not pregnant, and I still have the urge to chomp down on it.

My family keeps telling me to just give it a try, than maybe I will lose my obsession with wanting to eat it. For now, I will just keep chewing on Tums to try and curb my urge.

And just consider it one of the whacky side effects of the medicine . . . but if you should see me licking my lips around a chalkboard . . . now you'll know why!

10-1-09

Happy Pink Month

Hello Dears,

Today marks the first day of 2009's Breast Cancer Awareness Month. Now, being as that you are all on my "list", I can say w/o question, that you have all been "aware" of Breast Cancer over the last several months due to my story.

Never-the-less, I didn't want the day to go by w/o saying Happy Day! I continue to hope that by sharing my story with you, you in-turn share it with someone else, who then does the same. More and more people will know, and the more people that know, the more people will check their ta-ta's. And, the more people who check their ta-ta's, the more chances there are to catch the c-word early. I am here, doing well because of Early Detection, so keep passing the word along, and keep helping women find the c-word early until there is a cure.

I am in the "seventh inning stretch" right now and doing my best to be as comfortable as possible. I am done getting "filled" . . . thank GOD, because I really have no more elasticity in my skin. So Dr. Banbury is just allowing my body to get use to the size for 6 more weeks before she takes the expanders out!

I do have a surgery date for the "exchange" as they like to call it. I am scheduled to get my new silicone valley's on November 10th. It is an outpatient procedure, so all I need to do is show up, strip down, and finally get some sleep☺

Everyone that I have talked to, who has been through the procedure, has told me that this surgery is a lot easier to heal from than the mastectomies. So, I intend to be good and healed by Turkey Day!

I will be in touch once more before the surgery, but in the meantime . . . check your ta-ta's again, check your wife's ta-ta's again, tell your Moms, your Sisters, your Nieces, your Grannys, your Aunts, your Cousins, your Friends, your co-Workers, and your Neighbors, to check their ta-ta's too! . . .

Do it for me and for all of the other women who wear the Pink Ribbon Proudly.

My Love to You All,

Milinda

PS. one last note: I know that some of you are planning to participate in the upcoming Strides Against Breast Cancer Walk. That is fabulous! I will be there running with my Sister and Jason, and then walking. I will do my best to look around the crowd for familiar faces, but in-case I miss you, please know how personally thankful I am that you will be there to show your support for such an important cause. Next year, when I have more time to plan, I will set up a team so that we can all participate together. As for this year, I am just incredibly Blessed to be able to run it while "under construction".

THE BLANKET LETTER
TO MY SISTER ALISSA

And Hello,

If I had to describe you . . . my big sister—in one word, it would be . . . BLANKET.

Not only during the past few months, but over my lifetime, you have been my BLANKET.

Blankets are warm, they are soft, they are inviting . . . they seem to take care of you when you need them the most, and always wrap themselves around you with ease and grace.

Blankets always fit.

No matter what the weather outside, Blankets always make you feel sheltered from ALL that is going on in your life. Blankets are a sign of comfort, a sign of relief, a sign that your "moment" is over for the time being, and that you are "ok" to rest your weary head.

Blankets last a lifetime.

A true Blanket never strays, and is always there when you need to feel at peace and at home, no matter where you lay your head.

A good Blanket will embrace you when you are cold, when you are weary, when you are tired, when you are overwhelmed, when you are confused, when you are overjoyed, when you need it the most . . .

No matter how many miles separate you from those that you love . . . an exceptional Blanket, can reach across states. It can reach

---

across phone-lines, it can reach across fields, and roads that go on for miles an miles . . . across the universe and BEYOND.

A true BLANKET can do all of the above and more.

You are my BLANKET.

You always have been, and you always will be, no matter what. No matter what.

Thank You for being the best Big Sister in the entire world. Thank You for being my BLANKET.

I love you more than words can express. I love you like we love our warm, comfy, old and new Blankets.

Thank You for my treat week, and for ALL that was included in that long list of treats—from the tickets, to the exceptionally designed room, to the fun, fun clothes . . . and everything else.

Thank You for coming up to run the Breast Cancer Race with me . . . our first of many together for years to come. As if we wouldn't before, now we will run with more of an UMPH—Kick its Ass kind of attitude!

Thank You for all that you have done in the past over our childhood, and our lifetimes. And for all that you will do in the future.

The best thing that you can do for me . . . is to keep being my Blanket . . .

But moreover, keep taking the best care of yourself, your girls and your family . . . for they are my Blankets too, and knowing that you are caring for yourself, and them, makes me smile from PINK ear to PINK ear.

I love you,

Milin

Bye-Bye Bosu Balls!

Hello Dears,

As we round out (no ta-ta pun intended) Pink Month I wanted to be in touch and write a few words.

It has been a wonderful Month for me, and our family. After a "treat-week" of visiting down at my sister's (she totally spoiled me with some new shirts to fit over my ta-ta's), we headed into the month knowing how far we have come, and how lucky we all are.

I have run into some of you, and want to Thank You for your hugs of support . . . and for not freaking out too much when I grabbed your hands to feel my expanders. You really can't fully appreciate how hard they are, until you feel them firsthand . . . So, Thank You for feeling me up, and sharing in the joy☺

My sister and her girls came up to help me celebrate my Birthday and to run the race with us. Unfortunately, the weather wasn't the greatest . . . but we geared up, and ran the race together despite the wind and rain. I realize how much of an accomplishment it was to run given that my surgery was only four months ago, and given that the expanders are still in place. It was incredible to be there, running each step with Jason and Alissa on both sides of me—something that even I can't describe in words. I am thankful for the strength that I have been able to keep, build and gain. Most of that strength has come from you, my Dears, from my Husband and from Reagan Rose.

As I looked around at the start of the race, there where a few other women who ran with Survivor sashes on, and Pink t-shirts. And while it gives me comfort to know that I am not the only one, I still want and wish that no one else has to endure.

So, again, check those ta-ta's . . . Early Detection saves lives, it's as simple as that!

Today I had my first check-up appointment at the Oncologist office. The nurse practitioner did a full physical exam, went over my meds, and cleared me with a clean bill of health☺ I will see Dr. Wozniak for my next check up in January. I was humbled—to say the least—as I looked around the waiting room. My journey has been hard fought, but much less harsh than others who were there today. There SO needs to be a cure for this dreadful disease . . . one day there WILL be.

We will be leaving to visit with Alissa and her family tomorrow night, and will enjoy Halloween weekend down south. Reagan has had her list of who is to be what for quite sometime now. Lets hope we all live up to her costumed expectations.

Jason and I will be celebrating our 10th Anniversary on October 30th, so there has been, and will continue to be much to toast to this month.

I will be getting my lovely-lady-lumps on November 10th. The surgery will, once again, be at Wilm. Hospital, and is planned to start at 10:30. It is an outpatient procedure, so as soon as we are home, and able, I will be in touch to let you know that I am doing OK, and enjoying the softer side of things.

Thank You all, again for your support, your love, your kindness, your affection, your thoughts and your prayers. I am so lucky to have you all on my list of Dears, and so very lucky indeed to be here.

Keep the hugs and prayers coming, for me and for all of the other women affected by the c-word.

My Love To You All,

Milinda

This is a letter that I had written for Jason to read to the SWAT team. My husband is a member of the team, and we both feel as if they are our brothers in arms. To say that they had our backs during my ordeal, would be a gigantic understatement. I'd like to share this with you as an example that one's family can be made up of many different people . . . these SWAT members are now a part of mine.

STRENGTH . . . YES
I AM STRONG.

But stronger are the people who support me in the fight. I told Jason at the beginning of this journey, that I would much rather be the one w/ the c-word, than standing behind, supporting, and watching my loved one go through it.

Speaking of standing behind . . . that is what you all do—You are SWAT . . . You stand behind each other, on your way into eminent dangerous situations.

In my eyes, you are heroes.

You go into these situations like stealth bombers. You show up, do your job, wreak havoc, stand together, work together, and leave . . . most of the time w/ no Thank Yous . . .

You may think that your "work" as the team goes unnoticed, but I can tell you, that your wives, your children, your families, your friends, your neighbors and even your other co-workers are awe-struck, and know how seriously you take that work.

I would like to Thank You. Thank you all for standing behind Jason and myself during this journey. I am so fortunate, and continue to be acutely aware of how lucky I am. I feel safer knowing that you are all there for me, and our family.

I have told Mico this before, as well as Ryan, and I will share it with you now . . . Ryan is even more beautiful on the inside than she is on the outside. Her steps made a difference, and the support that you have shown, in my name is incredibly appreciated.

I will hug you all in person, as I see you, or as I meet you . . . and Thank You again.

. . . I have heard more than a few of you say "I would go through any door with him" . . . (referring to other members of the SWAT team). You did go through a door for me, on the day of the surgery, on the phone, over email, in person and so on and so on. And I rest easier knowing that we have your support.

I am also here to lend support, to you and yours. I am strong, I am able, I am here, and will continue to be here. So, that being said, please know that all you need to do is ask . . . and I will do my best to lend a hand. We all go through tough times, each one of us, so please know that we (the Atallians) are here for you as well, whenever you need us.

In the meantime, and until I see each one of you, I will keep up the good fight, I will stay strong, and I will be working on these new silicone-valley's of mine . . . and when our paths meet in person, my arms will be open-wide to give you a hug.

Thank you again for the donation to the Breast Cancer Walk.

Be safe,
Keep well,

Milinda

Ps. And whatever you do . . . don't scratch the LENCO!

11-9-09

Private Parts

Hello Dears,

I hope this email finds you all doing well, and breathing in the glorious fall air. I wanted to be in touch before I go in for my "Exchange Surgery" . . . such a funny way of saying . . . . Comfortable ta-ta's on their way! We will be headed into Wilm. Hospital around 8:30 on Tuesday and I expect to be home by late afternoon . . . or as Reagan would say. "When the moon comes up" ☺

I have felt much like a mannequin for the past 5 months. Not in a bad way, but much as if my ta-ta's weren't my own. I was busy dealing with the stretching, expanding and trying my best to keep myself in good shape as I enjoy doing. While they might have looked semi-"normal" outwardly, they haven't really felt like my own yet.

Tomorrow, I much expect for my new ta-ta's to become my own. I will go back to having private parts. And while I have enlightened some people by allowing . . . or rather insisting that some of you feel how hard the darn expanders were . . . I will relish in the fact, that I will no longer have them to educate everyone with!

I will have some new lovely lady humps ☺ Some new ta-ta's. Some new Private Parts . . . that will be just that for the rest of my days. Oh—they will be bigger than my old ta-ta's . . . that's for sure. And they will be different. But—My Dears—the same heart that has embraced all of your loving care and support will be right at home underneath them.

I have been forever changed by having had Breast Cancer, and I can honestly say . . . without question . . . that I am a better person, inside, and out for having gone through the last 6 months.

The "experts" say, that the term Survivor can't really be used in the true sense until one has reached the five year mark of being cancer free . . . but I say that's total and complete "B-A-L-O-G-N-A", as Reagan would sing . . .

Being a Survivor is finding the lump, it's not being afraid to make a big decision, it's for going through with that decision and fighting hard to get yourself back to good form . . . and it's for knowing how very lucky I am to be on this earth with my Family and Friends who have supported me the entire journey.

As I have said before, my journey is not yet over . . . I don't think anyone who has Cancer can say that their journey is, or ever will be over. But I can promise you this. I will continue to be positive, to take one day at a time, to be the best Mom, Wife, Sister, Daughter, Granddaughter, Niece, Cousin, and Friend that I can be. I will not sweat what I cannot control, or what is unimportant in our daily lives. And I will relish in the genuine and good people that we surround ourselves with.

Thank You again, for all that you have done for me, and for my family

I will be in touch soon after my surgery with a brief email, to let you know that I am OK, and that my new Ta-Ta's are finally in place.

Until then, keep me in your prayers, along with my family and the team of medical staff that will be helping me on Tuesday morning.

My Love To You All,
Keep Me,

Milinda

Decorations for our Christmas Tree

So, we are getting ready to leave for the exchange surgery. I was feeling a tad under the weather from a lovely sinus infection that was pending. The mood was somewhat tense, and I could feel my sister and Jason's united front, to remain strong and just get this over with.

I was putting on the robe that I wore to the hospital (if you ever need to have surgery on your chest, for any reason . . . I highly recommend wearing a robe—easier on and off), and Jason came in to take one last look at the expanders.

By this time, they were in my armpits, one was up higher than the other one, and one was closer to my inner chest than the other. Oh, I was a real looker at that point. Still, Jason took me in his arms and hugged me tight.

Then he whispered something into my ear to pass on to Dr. Banbury . . . he said, "Can you please tell Dr. Banbury that I'd like her to save the expanders so that we can use them as ornaments for our tree!" Is he a hoot or what—we laughed our way to the hospital!

Of course, I had to pass that along to Dr. Banbury as she was marking me up with a marker before I went under. She hadn't heard that one before, but I am sure she will pass it along to many of her patients to lighten the mood as they head into the OR.

Tis the Season to be Jolly . . . Ta-Ta, Ta, Ta-Ta, Ta-Ta!

Hello Dears,

I wanted to be in touch with you to let you know that I did well with the exchange surgery and, and I am on my way to recovering fully. The surgery was on time, and went seem-less-ly-so. Despite the fact that I showed up with the beginnings of a lovely sinus infection, Dr. Banbury hung some antibiotic on my IV, and did her thing!

It is hard to tell just how fantastic things are at the moment. I am still wearing the gorgeous polyester zip-up bra contraption that I will be sporting until I see her (Dr B) next week. But I CAN tell you, that things are oh-so-soft and cuddly! I have enjoyed sleeping on my side with out rocks in the way, and my skin has relaxed through my chest and armpits. I have gone back to the use of a regular pillow and will continue to take things slow and steady just as I always do.

My sister was in town for the procedure and assured me that things looked great before she left. This is how much she loves me . . . as if—my Dears—you didn't know already . . . She sat with Jason during the long morning at the hospital, she stayed here with us to make sure that I didn't do anything for the first few days . . . AND, when we took the drains out from the pain ball that I had strapped around me for a couple of days . . . she used her shirt to stop the drainage, until Jason ran in with some gauze . . . . Yup, she used her shirt! Now that shirt went immediately in the washing machine, but never-the-less, without even flinching, she took care of me and my drainage. That's how unconditional her love is for me. As is Jason's. I count my blessing's every single day to call them both my best friends.

So now, I will continue to heal, and wait for the next phase of things. I assume after I heal up and the scars are done healing, I will start to talk about the tattoo's . . . who would have thought?!

I want to Thank You, all of you again, for your acts of kindness, your thoughts, your prayers, your understanding and your support throughout this entire summer and into the fall. As we stand strongly on the verge of this Holiday Season, our family has so much to be Thankful for, so very much indeed. And you—my Dears—are on the list of Thanks and Praise!

So, if you hear me singing "Tis the Season to be Jolly . . . ta-ta, ta-ta, ta, ta-ta, ta-ta" . . . a little bit early this year, or if you hear me singing it throughout the year even after the holidays have come and gone . . . you can go ahead and let that smile creep across your whole face, enjoy the warmth of it, and consider it sent from me and my comfortable, soft, new, ta-ta's!

Keep checking yourselves and tell everyone that you love to do the same.

I will be in touch after a while, to let you know how things are going. Maybe not so frequently, but you will never be off of my Dears list . . . so that means you will never be far from me, no matter where I am.

My Love To You All,

Milinda

Happy Christmas . . .
the True Meaning of Pink

I am a Mom, I am a wife,
I live a very Happy Life.

I found a lump, I made a choice,
Off with their heads . . . I gained a "voice".

Through emails, I have kept in touch,
With you My Dears—its meant so much,

To have your prayers, and thoughts, and love,
And
~ open arms for me to hug.

I am OK, I kicked "its" ass,
There is no "c-word" . . . "this too shall pass".

So as you hang up your wreaths and bows,
Take some time for yourself . . . go ahead, strike the pose-

Check your ta-ta's, take your time, and just put on a smile,
Check your ta-ta's, feel em' up, it is very very well worth while . . . .

And if you ever think you can't,
Remember me, and ALL of my rants,

For you My Dears, CAN do things too,
We own the love and faith to prove . . .

That strength and pos-i-tiv-ity,
DO make a difference you will see,

Soooooooo

Raise a glass, and relax, as I make this Glam. Toast,
Merry Ta-Ta's to you, and to ALL you love most!
ps. . . .

Checkin' your ta-ta's is necessary . . . just think . . .

Because I did, I now know . . . the true meaning of PINK:)

1-27-10

Pepperoni Pieces

Hello Dears,

I hope that all of you enjoyed a wonderful holiday season with those that you love.

Our family had one of the best Christmas' to date . . . *Just a few* of the many highlights . . .

Once again, Santa paid a special visit to hour home. Reagan was awaiting his arrival at the front door as she listened to the siren come down the street. I cry every time—and thank my husband for indulging my childhood dreams with his transformation into St. Nick each year for our neighborhood.

We hosted a number of family gatherings at our home, and attended a lively gathering at Aunt Nancy's as well. Lis and her family came in (delayed . . . a while . . . but in) on Christmas Night. So, Reagan was ecstatic to have her cousins here for "Christmas Dinner"!

This year, more than ever, Reagan was elated to see each decoration, receive each gift, sing each song, and taste multiple cookies of the season. It was a true joy to watch Christmas come alive in her little eyes, and to see her bring happiness with each and every hug that she gave.

We took our annual Termini's trip with Dad and Susan, and also attended the Light Show at Macy's. It was hotter than a hairdryer in there, and we had to wait an hour or so to see the show, but Reagan lit up like a Christmas Tree when she saw the lights—and recognized the Ray Conniff (my favorite) versions of the songs!

We also took a ride on the Wilm. Western Railroad again while Lis was here. Reagan was beyond excited to be on the train with Mommom, Steve, the Manfredis and of course. Mommy and Daddy. Everyone seemed to enjoy the ride, although there weren't a lot of displays to see . . . and I do have to note that

I got a tinge of motion sickness on that thing. Hmm, I don't know if we will make that an annual occasion, but it was neat to be there in the moment.

We were honored to host my Granny and Poppop's Christmas Dinner here at our home, and for the first time in a long while, all of the family was here. All of their children, every spouse, every grandchild, and all 5 of the Bradley great-grandchildren were able to come. It was a fun day, and we hope to continue the trend in the years to come.

For those of you who were aware, and those of you who were not, my Granny's recent surgery went well. She is a Survivor twice over, and awaits more good new from the oncologist in the upcoming weeks. Please keep her in your prayers. You will often hear me refer to Marie and Paul as "My Granny" and "My Poppop" . . . for while I share them with ALL of their grandchildren, and great-grandchildren, I still feel as if they are "Mine" . . . that is a true testament to how much love and support they have given to the individuals in our family over the years. I love them a lot and have gained much strength and faith through their examples over my lifetime.

We had many memorable moments with all of our loved ones, family and beyond. It was special for me to be able to embrace everyone that I could, to show our appreciation for all of the support that we have been given over the last year.

On that note

. . . a brief update for you, My Dears.

Physically, I am doing well . . . and mentally too—Strength in Positivity! "It" seems surreal at times, but I continue to be aware of how lucky I am.

My scars have healed from the reconstruction and I am moving along with the "nips" . . . more on that in a moment.

There are still areas on my back that are tingly-numb. It only "hurts" when someone or something (like a tight jog bra) rubs or touches it. No pain, just a weird abrasive type of feeling.

The lymphadema that I was experiencing in my left hand continues to come and go. I have been stretching regularly to prevent the swelling and that seems to help. I don't expect that to ever totally disappear, so it's just something that I will get use to as time moves along.

It is weird to have the implants, but I am getting use to them. They don't really move around as if I would have gotten an augmentation without having had the mastectomies. I am assuming that its because they are in the pockets created by the "turtle shells"—needless to say . . . there's not a lot of jingling going on . . . which is fine with me. There is nothing like the real thing . . . but I am still amazed at how the Dr. made something out of nothing.

I get these very strange "phantom itches" . . . on my ta-ta's. I feel the need to itch, I feel itchy. I go in for the scratch . . . and I feel—*nothing*—because I don't have feeling in most of my ta-ta's. I have to say, it drives me a little batty at night. I do try to scratch the area, hoping that somehow signals from my "working epidermis" will let the non-sensational areas know that I am trying to alleviate the itch . . . but, so far, no such luck.

Outside of that, all in all, I am doing well, and moving along with great strength. I still miss the belly-sleeping but I am learning to adjust. The number of pillows (during sleeping hours . . . thanks Lis for the awesome plum-decorative-pillows) . . . has been cut in half, so at least we are less crowded while we rest.

I am enjoying my workouts with no issues and have started to lift some weights again, so I am thankful for being able to do that.

I did have a minor "scare" if you will over the Holidays. Thankfully, it was non-related to the c-word, but as my Survivor friends will tell you . . . every little ache or pain makes you think twice. Long story short . . . as if . . . I got to experience a totally random bleeding cyst that appeared out of the blue—parking itself on my right ovary. My OBGYN thinks the horrific day of pain that I had was due to some twisting that was also taking place. Lovely. Luckily, it untwisted, so the pain subsided after a couple of days. That lead me to have an ultrasound . . . which confirmed the cyst was there and had to come out. Sooo. I had MORE outpatient surgery a couple of weeks ago to do just that. It was laperscopic and all is fine . . . just some soreness and a few small scars.

I keep telling my loving husband to "just consider my body to be the legend of a map . . . that also leads to my nether-regions☺" . . . I love you Babe! True love does conquer all. I was fortunate enough to have found it young, and continue to bask in it every day that I spend with my husband. (sniff sniff)

I saw Dr. Wozniak (my oncologist) in mid-January and he gave me a 6 month, clean bill of health☺ I will see him again in three months for another check up. I am still taking the Tamoxifin, which seems to be OK . . . the hot flashes are still HOT . . . but nothing that I can't handle.

So, at this point, you must be asking yourself . . . what's up with the Subject Line . . . right?! Well, My Dears, that would be my husband . . . once again, making me laugh through it all.

It's kind of hard to imagine "nips" now that I have been living "plain" for 7 months. I forget what my old ones looked like, how big they were, etc. . . All I know is that somehow, despite my small size, I was able to feed my girl for a year out of those teeny things, which is still amazing to me. When Jason and I were talking about my upcoming appointment with Dr. Banbury, we wanted to go to the appointment with some sort of idea as to how we could determine size, shape, color, etc. . .

We tried dimes (too small), quarters (too small), 50 cent pieces (still a tad too small) . . . keep in mind that while my new ta-ta's aren't the biggest ones around . . . they are in-fact bigger than my old set . . . so this was all a bit perplexing. At last, Jason comes out with . . . "Babe, how about Pepperoni?".

Needless to say, he's about right! The appointment for my tattoo's is on May 27th so, I will bring along a few pieces for Dr. Banbury to use as a reference!

So, in a nutshell . . . there's the latest~ never a dull moment in the Atallian abode.

I am 8 or so months out since the "discovery" and doing well. I continue to be humbled by all of the well wishes that we have received along the way, and will continue to be grateful each and every day of my life that I am healthy, happy and here.

To have your support, thoughts, prayers, and hugs, not only for me, but for husband and Reagan as well, means the world to us. I am so very lucky. I can only hope that you too receive the kind of affection and loving expressions in your everyday lives that I am fortunate enough to receive in my world.

Reagan and I are headed to South Carolina this weekend (Jason has to work ☹), to help celebrate Bailey Rose's 6th Birthday! To see the girls (Mackenzie, Bailey and Reagan) play and enjoy being together makes my heart fill with joy each and every time.

I will be in touch again, to let you know how the "Pepperoni" turns out. I will continue to enjoy each and every moment that I get to spend surrounded by a healthy life and happiness.

Until I type again—check those ta-ta's. I have met so many Survivors that have beat their c-word because of early detection . . . so get to squeezing . . . then order a pepperoni pizza and think of me☺

My Love To You All,

Milinda

3-25-10

$$10 + 9 + 4 + 13 = 36$$

Hello Dears,

~A little math for everyone to give your minds a work out.

I hope this email finds you in a Spring state of mind. I will go onto explain myself as time is precious . . .

10 months since my "discovery"
9 months since my mastectomies
4 months since my reconstruction
13.1 miles I ran with my sister last weekend in the CR
=
36 . . . B . . . :0)

and a lil'—that's about what size I am touting around these days . . . so I thought it added up for me to be in touch.

My sister came into town for her Birthday weekend, and (for the second year in a row) we ran every single step of the Ceasar Rodney half marathon together. I wish that I could tell you that it was an easy race, but that just wouldn't fit my mold now would it?! I was fresh off a Spin Instructor Certification course from the weekend before and had a certain "tweak" in my knee that made itself known from about mile 4 til' the end of the race. If it weren't for my sister, I don't know if I would have pushed myself through. But, Lis was there with me from the start, encouraging me to keep going, no matter how slow I needed to run.

The thing that was magical for me about this race, despite the hard run, was that all along the course, we saw everyone that I hold closest to my heart.

Lis ran it with me . . . big sister, best friend—nuff' said.

Jason and Reagan were the first smiling faces we saw as we shredded our shirts and headed into the hills.

You couldn't help but hear the train whistle in the distance, so it was only a matter of time before Lis spotted Dad and Susan hanging out in front of their abode, train-whistling as we went by. My Dad had been in the hospital the week before with a bad infection that took a while to get under control, but still he stood out there . . . pic line and all, cheering us on.

As we made our way up to Kentmere Parkway, I saw a vision I will never forget . . . . My Granny, My Poppop and My Mom were all there, arms raised, cheering for us . . . of course, we stopped for a much needed kiss and hug.

We ran on, and once again, saw my two greatest gifts, Jason and Reagan posted up outside of the Art Museum.

After finishing up the hills . . . at least all but the last one . . . we once again, heard the train whistle on our way back down the Brandywine . . . Dad and Susan were still there waiting for us to run by again.

And, last but not least, as Lis and I made our way up the long, steep, seemingly never-ending hill that dawned the FINISH LINE sign on the tippy-top . . . we saw, and heard, Jason, Reagan Rose and my Mom, smiling from ear to ear, cheering for Lis and I, crying with tears of pride as we crossed the finish line hand in hand.

It wasn't my best time minute-wise for a race . . . as a matter of fact, it was my worst . . . but that doesn't really matter. I was there, in the moment, running for ta-ta's with my sister, being cheered on by ALL of the people who I love most in this world. Thank you to my wonderful family. I love you so.

Regardless of what age I am, or what it is that I am doing—to have my Husband and Daughter, as well as my Parents, and Granny & Poppop there supporting Lis and I, is something that I will not and do not take for granted. It's something that I strive for—to make them proud of me with *all* that I do.

Once again, I will say. I am so very lucky, to be healthy and here in these wonderful moments that make up my life.

So, My Dears, I hope that you surround yourself with those that are genuine, those that you love and those that love you back. Set your goals—whatever they may be—and then realize that anything is possible with strength and positivity.

For those of you that have asked, and I so appreciate it, my Granny is doing well. She is recovering from her node-removal surgery and has started to take her meds . . . which is the only treatment she will need. She is a strong woman, full of Faith, abundantly loved and admired, as is my Poppop, and we will continue to cherish our time with them each and every chance we get.

—

I will be in touch again soon, as I head into the Doctor's office for some tattoo work in mid April. Dr. Banbury asked me to bring a couple of slices of pepperoni with me . . . oh my.

Until then, we will be going on about our daily routines, while soaking up spring. Reagan will be starting her Kickaroo soccer and continuing with her swim lessons, and Jason will start his training for the three Triathlons that he will be doing over the summer months.

And now onto the least self indulgent part of this email—what I'd like you to do, is—open a window . . . let in some spring air . . . pour yourself and yours a glass of vino . . . turn on some Andrea Bocelli . . . or U2 . . . or whomever it is that "does it for you" . . . pull up your shirt . . . take off that bra . . . and get to squeezin' . . . start off your night with some **ta-ta** time. Check yourself out, and have your "other" do the same. And then go back to your glass of vino, and your music, and do whatever else it is that you may feel like doing ☺!

My Love To You All,

Milinda

No Pa-diddles Please

I feel as if now would be a good time to revisit the nips. Originally, I opted for a right nipple save. My initial thought was that I could hang on to my right one, because it was on my healthy ta-ta. I thought that Dr. Banbury could use it to match the other side with, when it came time to rebuild my left nip.

After thinking it over, and living with my new ta-ta's, I decided against using my old nip. For one, I didn't want to have a permanent set of high beams. And, secondly, while I know how fantastic Dr. Banbary is at her craft, I didn't want to end up with anything remotely resembling a pa-diddle (one high beam, and the other . . . well, not a high beam).

So, that is why, after a little thought and a little livin' with my new set, I decided to forgo the nipple saving and rebuilding process. and just go with the tattoo's.

For if there is one "plus" about having mastectomies and reconstruction, it's that I never have to worry about my high beams poking out to say—hello!

TA~TA TATTOOS

Hello Dears,

Well, after yesterday, I can no longer say that I am an ink-virgin!

For some reason, I was very nervous about getting my tattoos. Perhaps its because I was not going to be "under" for it, or maybe because somehow I thought I would feel it, or it could have been because it was yet another step along my c-word journey.

Whatever the reason, I was nervous going in. But, Dr. Banbury and I have a great relationship, so she immediately put my mind at ease and assured me that I would be just fine.

There is a needle that she could have given me to get my ta-ta's numb, but since I don't get numb for dental fillings (yes, I am one of those people) and since I don't have much sensation in my ta-ta's, we decided to go for it without the numbing medicine. And, it was as she said . . . just fine. I didn't feel much of anything except for the occasional twinge here and there. I am sore and tender today, but that will subside.

We picked out some colors, figured out a size (very much like a slice of pepperoni), and got started with artwork! It took about two hours from start to finish, but about an hour and a half for the actual tattoos.

It's amazing how many shades of pinks and browns there are, but we seem to have settled on a good hue and will re-evaluate in about a month. She wanted to go a tad lighter to begin with because it's much easier to add to, to make them a little darker. They will fade a bit, so that is another reason why she is going to take a look in about a month and most likely add some more pigment.

It was a bit of an outlandish feeling, to be lying there having nips tattooed on my chest, but I continue to count my blessings each and every day, and realize how fortunate I am in every moment.

As I shared with you before, Lis and I ran the CR half marathon together in March . . . whew that was tough this year!

I ran another half marathon last weekend in Lewes by myself. Jason and Reagan were there for support, of course—my biggest and best cheerleaders. The run was beautiful. Half of it was on trails, and the weather was perfect. Though I missed my sister immensely, it felt awesome to be out there having a good run.

Lis is going to come up, once again, in May to run another half marathon with me in Wilmington . . . this one should not be as hilly as the CR ☺!

Reagan is still enjoying her swim lessons and has started to play soccer on Saturday mornings as well. She's a natural. We are still very pleased with St. Mary's. Her teachers are wonderful and its been fun to see Reagan developing relationships with her classmates (more on that next Hello Dears). She will be going there again next year in the Three Day—Three Year Old Program.

Jason has started his training for his Tri's (his first of three races will be on Memorial Day weekend down in Sea Isle) and is still busy at work. I guess crime never sleeps! He will be attending another SWAT school in a week or so down in Charleston.

We continue to enjoy spending time together and watching Reagan as she grows into a lovely, lively, little girl.

One day, she will understand all of "this" and will surely be able to smile, laugh and cry through it all, as we have.

I will be in touch soon to let you know how the ink is holding up . . . for now-

-As the days move through the spring, we will soon be nearing Mother's Day. Surely, this year will be even more meaningful to me.

Its a fact: all of our Mothers are/were women. And whether you may be a Mother yourself, or perhaps a Mother figure to someone in your life, there is no denying that we were all nourished to life by women. Undoubtedly, all of these/those women had ta-ta's . . . so along with hugging your Mother, or a woman who may feel like a Mother to you, or a Dear friend, encourage them and yourself to ~

CHECK YOUR TA-TA's ☺! Check them in the car, in the kitchen, in the bathroom, in the shower, in bed, on the couch, in line at the grocery store . . . its possible . . . just check them, for me and for you!

My Love To You All,

Milinda

"TA-TOO-TOO-TOO, TA-TA-TA-TA, THAT'S ALL I WANT TO SAY TO YOU" . . . .

Hello Dears,

One the eve of this years Mother's Day, I wanted to be in touch.

I did something yesterday that was a little hardcore ☺ so, of course, I have to share it with you.

I got inked! Yup that's right! I'll get into the ta-ta tattoos in just a moment. But, I got myself a bon a fide, bodacious, beautiful tattoo.

It is a Pink Ribbon. Very eloquently and tastefully done. It's somewhat 3D-like, because of the shading that the artist used. I love it already and know it will look even more spectacular when it is healed.

Now, for the placement . . . I have been thinking of getting the ribbon for a while now, and I always knew where I'd like it to go. It's on the back of my left ankle.

My left side, because, that is the side that the "c-word" was on. The ankle, because its part of my body that I use to run and move forward. Also, I wanted the ribbon to be behind me.

I have no delusions that Breast Cancer will ever not be a part of what has made me, me. But, I am glad that these parts of it(the last almost twelve month parts) are behind me . . . and I intend to keep it that way.

Thus, the ribbon is a part of me, but behind me, on the very thing that I use to propel myself ahead each and every moment.

It hurt like the dickens, I am told because I happen to choose an area surrounded by tendons and bone. Ouch! I kept telling myself, "Milinda, you can do this, look at what you've done with your ta-ta's, you can totally get this Pink Ribbon" . . . and I did . . . so fun!

I know that tattoos aren't everyone's cup of tea, and that's OK. But I am happy to have been inked, especially on the verge of this Mother's Day, as its something that I will remember forever.

OK~ . . . . "now you see'um, now you don't" . . . .

As for the ta-ta tattoos, well that's a whole different monster.

Dr. Banbury somewhat warned me that they would fade a bit after I had them done. They lasted about 7 days at the most! I am serious! If you were to take a gander at them now (no worries, I will NOT be flashing anybody), they would just look like part of my scars from the mastectomies. It all blends right on in!

So, I called her office and told them of the travesty and she is ordering a new machine. We will see how this shakes out. I am willing to try one more time, to see if she can get them to "take" to my skin. Obviously, they use a different machine than the gentlemen at Monster Tattoo shop. Whatever machine she was using, is not working, so she is going to call me when the new one comes in and we will try again. The ta-ta stories are never-ending are they not?!

It's hard to complain about a little fading when everything else is so wonderful. We live a happy life here at the Atallian abode. I love being a Mom more than anything I've ever done. So, I am honored to be able to enjoy Mother's Day this year in a healthy, happy and loving state of mind.

You know where this is going right . . . . Get your squeezing digits out. Call your Mom, your Sisters, your Aunts, your Cousins, your Friends and Neighbors, your co-workers, your Mentors, your peeps at the Gym, whomever you care about that has ta-ta's . . . call them and tell them . . . "its that time again" . . . Milinda said to grip and grab, squeeze and squinch, kneed and knuckle, do whatever you need to do, but check those ta-ta's. And have an awesome Mother's Day.

My Love To You All,

Milinda

FATHER'S DAY

June 20, 2010

Dear Jake,

On Fathers Day this year, I wanted to take a moment to say a few things to you, my husband.

We have had one hell of a year to say the least. Though I will try through the lines in this letter, I don't think there are enough words that could describe what you've done for, and meant to me, and to Reagan over the past twelve months.

I said in the beginning of this c-word journey of ours, that I would much rather be the one battling, than you, or any other immediate family member of mine. I can't fully imagine what it must have felt like to be the one supporting me, and not the one going through it. Selfishly, I don't ever, ever want to know.

The love, strength, optimism, encouragement and unwavering kindness that you have given me, have helped me be as steadfast as I have been.

That is what you are to me: you are my **strength**.

Strength can be defined in many ways, but you my dear encompass them all for me. You are foundationally strong. You are mentally strong. You are emotionally strong. Your character, ability and will, are strong in everything you do. You are supportively strong. And, as if it wasn't obvious to anyone that sees your handsome physique, you are most definitely physically strong as well. All of these strengths have been with me over this past year. Even when you weren't trying, with your strength behind me and beside me, I knew that everything was going to be OK.

I promise to keep trying and to keep doing, every single day. I will never give up on anything that is important to you and to our family. I will stay strong because you are by my side. Being the best husband, my best friend, and most of all, the best Dad to our Reagan Rose.

Everything else, everything else in this world is secondary.

So, on this Fathers Day, I want to say, thank you . . . thank you for picking me almost 19 years ago, thank you for wearing the Pink ribbon, thank you for going to my Dr.s appointments with me, thank you for sitting in the hospital waiting rooms while I had my surgeries, thank you for covering my ass as I made my way across the hallway the night of my mastectomies—and for laughing with me after my bodacious burp, thank you for taking care of me when I was recovering, thank you for not letting me push myself too hard, thank you for laughing through our tears with me, thank you for all of the hilarious nicknames that you called my expanders, thank you for talking to your friends at work about what we were going through, thank you for sheltering me and our family from issues that are not important to us, thank you for being proud of me, and for saying just that—I strive for that every day, thank you for coming to all of my races and for cheering loudly with Reagan, thank you taking the time to take care of yourself—you know that makes me happy, thank you for still thinking that I am beautiful and for loving the woman that I am today, thank you for holding my hand, and thank you for being such a wonderful Daddy to our Reagan Rose . . . because that's what its all about.

Happy Fathers Day, I love you so very much.

Your Wife,

Milinda Rose Atallian

June 26, 2010

Pinkalicious

Hello Dears,

Well today is the day. It has been one full year since my mastectomies. In my mind, that makes me a one-year Survivor! YIPEEEEE!

So many things have happened over this past year. I can honestly say, without a doubt, that for me personally, most of those things have been fantasticly fabulous ☺.

Having Breast Cancer has changed my life in many ways: physically, mentally, spiritually, emotionally, and beyond.

The love, affection, attention, appreciation, and genuine acts of kindness that have been bestowed upon myself, and my family are indescribable. To be able to connect, and reconnect with members of our family, as well as neighbors—whom we now consider to be family, and friends, has just made this whole experience one that I am grateful for. Yup, I said grateful for.

It may sound strange to some, but having the "c-word", and being able to overcome it, is something that I am grateful for.

"It" has shown me what the meaning of true is. True strength, true love, true support, true dedication, true frustration, true inspiration, true tears, true laughter, true family, true friends . . . this list could go on and on.

In my humble little Milinda opinion, to be true to someone and something is to give it your utmost, genuine, presence and energy—to give it all that you can, and never let up—not today, not tomorrow, not ever.

And, so I promise to be true to the effort that I will continue to fight. I will **fight on** because I know that my battle will never truly be all the way over. I will continue to be true to my family and those that we love and care about.

There have been many highlights, or dare I say, peaks and valley's (that pertain to my ta-ta's) over the past year . . . I will put all of them in a safe place and share them with you when the time is right, so please make some room on your nightstand and your bookshelves for that :0) . . .

Our trip to Kiawah this year was fantastic. No stress, no worries . . . just everyone hanging out and enjoying the moments. Time flies by so quickly. Soon enough Reagan and my neices will be sunbathing on the beach, instead of letting the sun kiss their bodies as they play in the sand. My sisters girls and Reagan are building a bond that will surely last a lifetime. The nostalgia that I feel when I watch them enjoying each others company is amazing. I have been so lucky to have made such wonderful memories with my family over my lifetime, our foundation is strong and will remain so.

Jason's triathlon in Charleston was awesome . . . it was hot . . . like standing in an oven, but I will always remember what he said to me as he cooled down after the finish . . . "It was so hot that I wanted to walk, but I looked down at my pink ribbons on my bike, and my pink bracelet and thought . . . if my baby can run three half marathons w/in a year of kicking the c-word's ass, then I can keep going". So he did, he kept going and turned out his best personal time thus far in his triathletic career. He is such a strong man, strong in every sense of the word.

Hearing him say that is part of the many reasons as to why I have shared so many things from this past year. If I can motivate someone to keep going . . . keep moving forward . . . keep taking care of themselves, no matter what, **no matter what** . . . then I have done what I have set out to do . . . that—and to have you all squeezin' your ta-ta's.

As I stood at the foot of the ocean in Kiawah yesterday after my run, the very same ocean that I stared across last summer, I let the tears fill my eyes and I filled my lungs with the ocean breezes. In and out, in and out . . . just like the waves that lapped the shoreline. There are many things that are connected together by the ocean . . . . With that in mind, I kept breathing deeply and cast out all of the true emotion, the true love, and the true appreciation that I hold in my heart for all of you ~ My Dears.

I re-dedicated myself to the notion to live strong and in the moments. To not waste time or energy on things that are not important to our family and those that we love most. And to be thankful for the time that we spend togehter with little worry and no stress. Life is too precious to live it any other way.

Somehow, someway, wherever you are—whether it be today, or in the days ahead, the next time you touch your toes to the ocean waters, you will feel me. You will feel my thanks. All you have to do is take a moment to breath, close your eyes, picture me with my Pinkalicious (one of Reagan's favorite books) smile, and know how thankful I am to have you in my life.

I am a happy wife, a happy mother, a happy daughter, a happy sister, a happy aunt, a happy sister in law, and on and and on and on. I am happy and healthy . . .

I am here, and I am OK now.

I will be in touch from time to time, so that I can remind you and yours to check your ta-ta's. I want to Thank You for sharing your time, your minds, and your thoughts as you read over the happenings of my fight against the c-word this past year. Jason, Reagan and I will be forever grateful, and will continue to greet you all with open arms when we are in your company.

Keep feeling those ta-ta's. Tell everyone that you love to do the same. Share my story with them and tell them the same thing that the Dr. told me on the day that I found out I had Breast Cancer . . . "you have saved your own life".

I did it. You can do it. It can be done.

My Love to You All,

Milinda

TA-TA

And so, this is the story behind my journey, or at least my journey up until now. There are a few reasons that I wanted to put my Hello Dears in book form—I think its important to share them with you now.

First and foremost, since my daughter was two when I was diagnosed, and is now rounding out her third year, I wanted to have something in writing that she can read when she is mature enough to handle "knowing". Knowing that her Mom had Breast Cancer, and how I went about kicking it's ass!

I want Reagan to have something that she can read, and then pass along to her children, should she be blessed enough to have them someday.

I want her to know that I did kick "it's" ass, and that part of my strength came from being her Mommy. I want Reagan to know that I will continue to fight, for the rest of my life, so that maybe one day others won't have to. I want my daughter to know that laughter through tears is one of the best things in this world.

I can only hope that she is one day as proud of me, as I am of her and my husband, for going through this journey with me.

The second reason is simple. Some of my Hello Dears requested that I write this book. Keeping in touch with them, and sharing my journey with them has been part of my treatment.

For me, knowing that my Dears could worry a little less, because they knew what was going on, was very important. I want them all to be able to remember, when they see the pink cover of this book on their bookshelves, that they were a part of something special . . . and that they should check their ta-ta's again and again!

Lastly, I want everyone who opens the pages of this book to know that forward motion is what you need when you are faced with anything that is less than fantastic.

Keep moving forward.

That will mean something different for each of you, and that is OK. I have been asked time and time again, "How are you still smiling? How are you still OK?"—Two words, forward motion.

I know that my journey will never be over. I continue to deal with all that a Breast Cancer diagnosis and treatment has to offer for someone of my age. It is hard, and it is work, everyday it is work. But, I keep moving forward so that I can look back on what I have done and accomplished along the way.

For me, forward motion is moving from one thing to the next. Doing my best to take care of one thing, and continuing on to the next thing. There is no wasting of precious time feeling sorry for myself. Forward motion means taking care of myself, so that I can take the best care of the people that I love the most. It means continuing to uphold and build traditions that are so near and dear to my heart, with my family. Forward motion is what helps me motivate those that I love and those that I surround myself with, to make them better every day—to try and be present in the moments.

Forward motion is what has gotten me to this point, and will continue to fuel the current that will keep my motion perpetual for the rest of my days.

Positivity, strength, faith, friendship, loyalty, patience, appreciation, admiration, emotion, empathy, thoughtfulness, trueness and genuineness, laughter and love, these are the words that I have learned the profound meaning of throughout my journey.

I will continue to encourage and hope that everyone, young and old, check their ta-ta's on a regular basis, so that they too can save their lives, as I did mine. ta-ta ~

Author's Bio

My name is Milinda Rose Atallian. I was 34 years old when I was diagnosed with Breast Cancer. I have been blessed with the most supportive parents, as well as a big sister, whom I consider to be my best girlfriend. I was lucky enough to marry my high school sweetheart, and together we share a beautiful daughter named Reagan Rose. I enjoy being a stay at home Mom, as well as taking good care of myself by running and teaching Spinning. I am a happy wife, mother, daughter, sister and friend to all that I share my life with.

www.ingramcontent.com/pod-product-compliance
Lightning Source LLC
Chambersburg PA
CBHW020351290526
45785CB00005B/2231